How to Understand and Deal with Stress

Katy Georgiou

T0190782

The Experiment, LLC
220 East 23rd Street, Suite 600
New York, NY 10010-4658
theexperimentpublishing.com

This book contains the opinions and ideas of its author. It is intended to provide helpful and informative material on the subjects addressed in the book. It is sold with the understanding that the author and publisher are not engaged in rendering medical, health, or any other kind of personal professional services in the book. The author and publisher specifically disclaim all responsibility for any liability, loss, or risk—personal or otherwise—that is incurred as a consequence, directly or indirectly, of the use and application of any of the contents of this book.

The Experiment's books are available at special discounts when purchased in bulk for premiums and sales promotions as well as for fund-raising or educational use. For details, contact us at info@theexperimentpublishing.com.

Library of Congress Cataloging-in-Publication Data available upon request

ISBN 979-8-89303-026-6
Ebook ISBN 979-8-89303-027-3

Cover and text design by Summersdale Publishers

Manufactured in the United States of America

First printing September 2024

Contents

Introduction

Stress is a natural reaction to the highs and lows of life. Life throws us curveballs and stress is our body's response. We don't have to fear it, but it doesn't have to consume us either. In small doses, stress can spur us on to keep pushing and reaching our goals. In large amounts it can slow us down, or over time become chronic, affecting our physical, emotional and mental health.

In the following pages, you'll find tips for navigating your stress when it all gets to be too much. Part 1 explains the science of stress, helping you identify your personal triggers, spot early signs and keep ahead of the game to buffer the storm when life gets tough. Part 2 provides practical, creative ways to see you through to the other side. We can't always avoid stress but, if we understand it better, we can learn to work with it.

Understanding Stress

Stress is felt physically and emotionally. How much stress you experience and the way you respond to it depends on many factors, including what you're currently dealing with, past life events and the people who've influenced you. That's to say, everybody's going to feel and deal with it differently. Let's call this your life template. To tackle stress, you need to get to know your life template, so you know what you're dealing with. This chapter will help you understand your template and identify how stress shows up for you, giving you the science, reasons and triggers behind it.

Find your template

Grab some paper and pens. Draw a big circle and in the middle write everything that you have on your plate right now. To the left of that circle, sketch a quick time line of your life with key stressful events plotted in. To the right of the circle, write down the names of the people who were around you during these times in your life. Highlight those you remember turning to for help. You'll get a good visual picture of your life template: what's happened, who was there for you, where the bottlenecks of stress were and what you did about them. This can be a powerful way to see how much you're carrying with you and where you might need more support. For example, maybe there were very few people you could turn to during times of stress. If that's the case, notice how this makes you feel. Try showing your template to a trusted person if you feel safe enough, as they might spot some different patterns.

Know yourself

Your chances of feeling stressed will increase in times of transition or change, like moving house, leaving a job, losing someone you love, if you're under pressure or dealing with many things at once. Sometimes stress can feel present even without a clear cause. When you're feeling this way, it can be useful to look back on your life and assess the stresses of your past. How did you deal with them? How did people around you deal with stress? Doing an audit like this initially can help you make sense of some of your patterns and where they came from. This can be brainstormed in your head, but be creative if you wish. Draw a time line of key life moments or play the songs you listened to in your youth —what do they conjure? What was going on in your life then?

Know your Fs

Many people are aware of the fight-or-flight response: it's the primal response to danger activated in times of stress that prompts you to flee or combat a situation for survival. But there are actually five Fs: Fight, Flight, Flop, Freeze and Fawn. Each of these is described in more detail on the following pages. Your reaction depends on many factors, including what you did in your very early development in response to being frightened. Research shows that whatever we did the first time to keep ourselves safe from danger gets hardwired into the part of the brain called the amygdala—that's the primitive part of our brain that we short-circuit to in times of trouble. That's why it can sometimes feel like our responses are out of control. The good news is, it doesn't have to stay that way.

Identify your stress responses

- Fight—you push back, get angry or try to defeat the thing that's overwhelming you.

- Flight—you avoid a situation, run away or retreat to escape the source of danger.

- Freeze—like a deer in headlights, you feel paralyzed. This can happen when escape isn't possible, because running may lead to a chase or fighting back risks more attack.

- Flop—this is a complete body collapse when muscles become floppy. You might faint, feel dizzy or experience dissociation. This usually happens when just freezing isn't enough to stop the source of stress. It is a common reaction for people who have experienced trauma. If that's you, there are plenty of tips in this book to help.

- Fawn—this is when you move closer to the source of danger, because appeasing an attacker or making friends with them is your best chance of staying alive.

We see evidence of these responses in the wild. Next time you watch a wildlife documentary, see how many you can spot. Depending on what's happened in your life, you may have done one or more of these things in reaction to stress. It's important to remember we aren't always in control of how our stress response shows up. Understanding this process can help you recognize that it's not your fault—it's actually your body's innate way to try to keep you safe which, in most cases, no longer serves you if you're not in danger any more. The examples on the following pages may help you better understand the type of stress response you have.

Fight response

You see a young child wander into a busy road. Without thinking, you grab the child and bring them to safety, maybe even putting yourself in harm's way. Your response can feel primal and automatic with a strong surge of emotion and energy. In a work situation, a tight deadline approaches, which gets your adrenaline pumping. The pressure to finish helps spur you on. In relationships, you say what's on your mind and expect the same back. Arguments don't scare you and you find it frustrating if a partner tries to smooth things over too soon. When you meet your match, you feel energized and pumped up. The fight response feels visceral. Your thoughts take a back seat as blood rushes to your head and your heart rate increases. You feel more tense than usual and it can take a while for what's happened to really sink in.

Flight response

You're late for an important meeting and start to sweat. You visualize everyone staring at you as you enter. The thought is too much, so you panic, flee the situation and don't turn up. Perhaps when you're taking an exam, you get up and walk out halfway through because you anticipate failure in advance. You retreat from relationships if things feel challenging and you'll walk away from conflict. Problems don't feel like challenges to be tackled, but obstacles to be avoided. You feel smaller and more vulnerable, tight in your chest and gut, and instinctively want to back away. You might notice yourself actually taking a step backward, recoiling or picture yourself running away. You're very aware of the exit signs in an enclosed space and might even figure out your escape routes in advance.

Freeze response

A car comes toward you and you can't move for terror. Or you're performing on stage and your mind goes blank, even though you know your lines well and have rehearsed them before. At work, you feel so overwhelmed with how much there is to do, you can't do anything at all. In this state, you can't make any decisions and can't ask for help because you don't know what to ask for. It can feel like you're glued to the ground. It can also feel like all your senses are blocked: you can't speak, hear or feel things. Your throat can become dry, as if your voice has disappeared. It's like your energy is locked inside of your body with no way out.

Flop and fawn responses

Flop: One moment you're fine, then suddenly you realize you've blacked out. On a smaller scale, your mind goes blank, you feel dizzy, confused or zone out easily. You might feel exhausted or like the shutters have come down. It can be triggered by feeling overwhelmed or an unpleasant memory. The effects can be delayed and a stressful day means you might sleep for a long time.

Fawn: You've already got too much going on, but if someone asks you for a favor, you take on the extra burden, usually at the expense of your own free time. This can make you prone to burnout. In a relationship, you go along with things, as the consequences of saying no feel more challenging than saying yes. With strangers you often override your instincts, like handing over money or getting in a car. You can often feel like you're running on autopilot.

Recognizing stress

Stress can be a response to an obviously important task, like taking an exam or preparing a presentation. Or it can be a response to a series of smaller simple tasks that build up and accumulate with limited time available to complete them. In these cases, stress arises because of the importance you're attaching to the event or for the loss of control your situation brings.

Stress can also result from unexpected life changes, such as such as the loss of a job or loved one.. Even positive life-changing moments, which on the surface make us feel good, can cause stress. For example, you might plan to have a baby, feel incredibly in love or be excited for a big trip you have planned, but all of these still mean a big change, and when change is on the horizon our minds and bodies react.

The quality of relationships we have will also impact how we feel. A poor relationship with a partner, spouse, parent, sibling or colleague can be a huge factor for stress. The following pages will help you recognize how stress can show up in your life in both obvious and less obvious ways, and how you can start to deal with it in a healthy, balanced way.

Spot the signs

The World Health Organization (WHO) defines work-related stress as "a reaction people may have when presented with demands and pressures that are not matched to their knowledge and abilities and which challenge their ability to cope." Symptoms include headaches, heavy chest pain, irritable bowel syndrome (IBS) and mental health changes, such as anxiety, panic or low mood. Some reports show that half of all people who leave their job in Europe do so as a result of stress, and that extreme stress is behind 75 percent of doctor visits in the US. How symptoms show up differs for everyone. It's important to track what goes on in your body when you're feeling stressed, as these can be helpful markers. Get in the habit of scanning your body each morning. If your heart is beating quickly or a body part is giving you trouble, give it a voice: What is it saying? What does it want?

Emotional triggers

For many people, going through a major life change is a huge trigger. For others, it's about feelings of control. If you're the sort of person who can't bear feeling in limbo, then something like waiting for exam results or buying a house can be especially stressful. If routine gets you down, then scenarios that force you into a strict timetable can feel unbearable. Have a think about the kinds of scenarios that leave you especially stressed. Start to identify any themes or patterns that connect them. This way you'll start to anticipate the scenarios that might leave you stressed before they happen, and then you can take measured steps to reduce your stress levels.

Physical triggers

A key to understanding your stress is identifying your physical triggers. Start with your basic needs including hunger, sleep and temperature. Research suggests that 15 to 20 percent of people experience stress-related problems when they haven't slept enough, while other studies show that stress suppresses appetite. Knowledge is power when it comes to spotting what your body needs to function well. You might wish to start a diary, keeping track of how stressed you're feeling, what basic needs were met that day, along with what you ate or drank. If you're not stressed right now, look back at any moments when you were: Were you tired, hungry or hot? Did you have any go-to behaviors such as comfort eating or drinking caffeine or alcohol? Try to create a picture of what your stress symptoms look like and how you react to them.

Simple vs. complicated stress

Simple stress has a clear cause, a clear end and is time limited. You can usually spot what's caused the stress and notice symptoms disappearing soon after. For example, in the run up to an exam, you may feel nervous and tense, with a stomach ache. Once your exam is over, these symptoms disappear. Other examples of simple stress include getting stuck in traffic when you're late for a meeting or trying to move house. Once it's over, you feel a release.

With more complicated types of stress, the time you spend feeling stressed doesn't always match the circumstance you're in and there isn't always one identifiable cause. Maybe you wake up clenching your jaw, feeling on edge and reaching for a stress ball, even though you've got the day off or feel quite happy with your life. The pages below will tackle this.

Hidden signs

We're not always aware we're stressed. Stress can operate in the background as we're living our daily lives. This makes it easy to ignore or not notice the telltale signs that our bodies and moods are giving us. If you've been feeling angry for a long time or going through a period of low mood and depression, these can be less obvious signs of stress that we don't immediately recognize as stress responses.

We can actually be living with many ongoing problems that we don't immediately link to being stressed. Some examples include involuntary tics, insomnia, stomach issues like irritable bowel syndrome (IBS) and colitis, migraines, missed periods, weight gain, hives, rashes, hair loss and intrusive thoughts. These are all issues that can be triggered by bouts of stress or made worse in stressful moments.

It's quite common for stress to show up in the same parts of our bodies each time. For example, maybe your stress always shows up in stomach-related issues or through headaches or as a sinus infection. Take a moment to think about how stress usually shows up for you and where you hold tension in your body. As a helpful prompt, notice how your body feels right now. Where are you experiencing tension, aches and pains?

Change up

Stress isn't only related to big changes, such as starting a new job or having a child. Change can be subtle, like getting older or losing your eyesight. These are incremental losses over time that can creep up on you if left unnoticed. Because they're gradual, we can deny they're happening, but they play havoc with your mind in the background. Think of this like a computer updating while you're typing. That extra effort over time can be felt in your body as stress. Take a minute or two to reflect on some of the little changes currently happening in your life. It can be painful to acknowledge them, but try to sit with the discomfort and share it with friends. Sharing doubts and fears with the people we love can be a release, as we increase our support and learn we're not alone.

Know your needs

The psychologist Abraham Maslow created an important theory about our hierarchy of needs. The idea is we cannot pursue hobbies and interests or even think about leading meaningful lives unless our basic needs are met first. If you're living through a war or in poverty, for example, you're in survival mode and life will feel like you're treading water until you're safe enough to plan ahead. In Maslow's theory we need food and water first, followed by shelter and then a need to feel safe. That could be a roof over your head, a job or financial security. Only then can you think about friendship, love, a meaningful career, education and hobbies. Take a moment to recognize which level you're at. If you're trying to reach for higher goals when your more basic needs aren't yet met, this will increase your stress.

Assess your work life

So much of our life is spent working. Who you're working with, where and how can be just as important as the job you're doing. Studies show that your happiness in the workplace depends on how much control you feel you have. For some, the stability of a full-time job with clear hours and paid annual leave is important, while for others it puts limitations on them. Take some time to recognize which aspects of your work life are creating stress. Is it the workload, the people, the way you're managed or how you're working? Getting clarity on this can be a helpful start to know what to do about it.

Audit your relationships

Take a piece of paper and list any important relationships you have. Maybe you're a parent, you have a best friend or you're a manager. As you work your way through your list, ask yourself how satisfied you are in these relationships? What do you mean to these people? What role do you take up? Would you like anything to change? This exercise will get you thinking about the people in your life, how satisfied you are in your relationships and your patterns of relating to people. You might, for example, discover that in most of your relationships you're always the one who makes decisions or perhaps you're the one who follows them. Think about that and about that and how it contributes to your stress. Are any relationships missing that you would like to have in your life? This will help you spot some sources of stress lying just out of your awareness.

Trauma-related stress

If you've experienced a trauma or a series of traumatic events in your life, your stress responses may be more pronounced. This can be the case if you have a diagnosis of post-traumatic stress disorder (PTSD), work in the military, have suffered or witnessed physical or sexual assault, violence or rape, have been involved in or witnessed an accident, experienced a particularly difficult childbirth, lived through a natural disaster, or suffered emotional, physical or sexual abuse. In some cases, the reactions you have to situations, or triggers unrelated to these events, can feel disproportionate—almost as if you're back in the situation you were in when the trauma occurred. For you, it will be important to take extra measures for your self-care and if you find your reactions especially debilitating, seek out formal support from a professional (there are details in Part 2). The flop response (page 15) may be the one you most recognize and you certainly aren't alone. It might be helpful to remember that this reaction is your body's way of trying to keep you safe.

The science of trauma

When you go through a traumatic experience, your hypothalamus, pituitary and adrenal glands release hormones to prepare you for one of your five Fs. You can experience tunnel vision or things going in slow motion. At its extreme you might dissociate, which means your thoughts, feelings and memories disconnect, your body desensitizes from pain, and your mind and body feel very separate, as if they don't belong to you. You may even fixate on a detail around you like a painting or a piece of chewing gum on the floor. While this might feel scary at the time, you'll be surprised how many people experience this. Learning a few coping strategies, outlined in Part 2, can go a long way to reducing its impact on you.

Post-traumatic stress disorder (PTSD)

Between 10 and 20 percent of people who experience trauma develop post-traumatic stress disorder (PTSD). This is more complicated and serious than everyday stress. It occurs when the initial impact of a trauma continues to interfere with your life and ability to function long after it has happened. The National Institute of Mental Health suggests these symptoms usually show up within three months of the traumatic incident. Signs can include distressing flashbacks, feelings of terror about simple, everyday tasks, hopelessness and severe inability to function day to day. The following pages explain more about the symptoms and why this happens, but you should contact your doctor for support if you think this is happening to you.

Complex post-traumatic stress disorder (CPTSD)

If you've experienced repeated trauma throughout your life as a result of sustained neglect or abuse over time (physical, sexual, psychological, racial) or through a series of isolated traumas that have built up into one larger issue, you might be aware of complex post-traumatic stress disorder (CPTSD).

This kind of stress disorder can be more severe if your trauma happened early on in your life, if the perpetrator was a parent or caregiver, or it went on for a long time. It's quite common to feel shame or guilt, to fall into despair, to mistrust people and relationships, and to take risks with drugs, alcohol and your life.

Remember this isn't your fault and with expert support your life can improve. Be careful not to self-diagnose and if you think you have CPTSD, seek out a formal assessment from a psychiatrist.

Brain changes

Studies suggest that the part of the brain called the hippocampus is smaller in people with post-traumatic stress disorder (PTSD). When the hippocampus doesn't function properly, this stops trauma from being processed effectively. High levels of stress hormones released during the trauma can cause you to feel numb or hyper-aroused. Symptoms can include flashbacks, nightmares, and intrusive and suicidal thoughts. This is part of the body's natural response to the trauma. This doesn't mean you can't recover. With time and expert help, you can build peace of mind again. Specialized therapies, which we will discuss in Part 2, work very effectively with this kind of stress and for many people can help lead to full recovery.

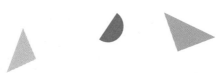

Types of stress

Stress can be acute, episodic or chronic. Acute stress is common to all of us and it happens in response to specific situations that startle, challenge or push us. It's usually quite harmless if a one-off, although if the situation causing acute stress is life-threatening it can lead to post-traumatic stress disorder (PTSD), as earlier described.

Episodic stress is a series of acute stresses that keep happening. This might occur if you're working in a high-intensity job or you're going through a big life change. If these levels of stress persist for long periods of time it becomes chronic stress, which impacts your body by weakening your immune system, increasing blood pressure and affecting your bodily systems. Once you're chronically stressed, it becomes easy to enter a cycle of destructive behavior. This may include turning to alcohol, eating more or skipping meals, consuming more sugar and salty food or smoking, which in turn further impacts your emotional and physical health. This is why it's so important to tackle it.

A stressed heart

Your adrenal glands release two stress hormones: adrenaline and cortisol. These increase your heart rate, which makes your blood pump faster and your blood vessels constrict to get more oxygen to the parts of the body that need to take action. This in turn increases your blood pressure. If your blood pressure is raised over a long period of time as a result of chronic stress, your risk of heart disease, stroke and heart attack increases. Don't panic, because these effects are reversible, and you can follow the tips in Part 2 to set you on the path to better health.

Stressed hormones

Stress can interfere with sexual libido and your ability to have sex. It can lower testosterone in men, cause erectile dysfunction or make menstruation more painful, heavier or irregular, affecting your ability to have children if you want them. If you already suffer from a condition like polycystic ovary syndrome, stress can make the symptoms worse.

A stressed gut

When you're stressed, you produce glucose from your liver, your stomach produces more acid and your bowel movements change, making you more likely to experience things like constipation, diarrhea, heartburn, acid reflux and nausea. Long term, this can place you at higher risk of ulcers or diabetes. Severe ongoing stress can sometimes trigger more chronic stomach problems like ulcerative colitis, which affects the bowel. But some lifestyle changes and professional help, along with meditative practice as outlined in Part 2, can work to ease symptoms.

Mental health

Stress levels and mental health are strongly connected. When you're stressed, you're less equipped to deal with life's mishaps. This can make you feel bad about yourself, cause a dip in your mood or lead you to become anxious and possibly depressed. In turn, these feelings can lead to further stress, which creates a vicious cycle. In moments of stress and periods of uncertainty, low moods can cause you to dwell on things, sometimes triggering intrusive thought patterns that become increasingly harder to dismiss. This is why it's important to seek help as soon as you can.

Self-assessment

Having read this far, notice the feelings you're left with and take a look back at the exercises you've done. What did you discover? Are you more or less stressed than you thought? After reading Part 2, you might want to come back to them and see if you notice a difference.

How to Manage Stress

Now you've understood your life template and triggers, the next step is knowing how to work with or manage them. This section will provide you with the tools to help yourself in times of stress, including practical and physical self-help tips to try at home, respected strategies from the world of therapy, along with medical and alternative health options. It will also show you who and where to turn to if you need more formal support or your feelings of stress are getting out of control.

What's on your plate?

In Part 1, you created a life template (see page 7). Take a look back at what was on your plate then. Have things changed? Make some edits to reflect where you are now. Notice how it feels in your body as you do this. If everything's the same, what does that do to you? Don't worry, this isn't a test and there's no expectation for you to be suddenly fine. If you're left feeling that nothing's changed or you still feel stressed, stay curious and look at why this is. It can take time to make sense of our experiences, so use this as an opportunity to tweak and experiment with any of the exercises and see what happens. Perhaps share your thoughts with someone you trust, and swap tips and ideas. Remember that you're the expert in your life, and this may give you another clue to what works for you.

Ground yourself

Contacting the ground is your first, baseline go-to response for stress and will be referred to throughout this section. It can be especially helpful if you find your stress regularly turns into panic. Wherever you are, whatever you're doing, place your feet flat on the ground so that you feel stable and close your eyes. If you're able to sit on the floor cross-legged or lie down flat, then even better. Think of this as earthing: really connect with the ground beneath your body. The following pages will teach you strategies to further ground yourself. Some studies suggest that this simple act can help reduce or relieve symptoms of stress such as pain and fatigue, reduce blood pressure and improve sleep. If you're feeling disconnected from the world, it can also remind you that you belong to it and you're a crucial part of it—the ground will always be there for you.

Feel the earth

A really easy way to ground yourself is to walk barefoot. You can do this in your home, feeling the carpet beneath your feet, walk on grass, a sandy beach or in mud. Touching and holding plants can also keep you grounded. It could be as simple as surrounding yourself with flowers and plants, but holding some soil in your hands, smelling it and getting a feel for its temperature and texture can really help. If you have time and space, you might even try planting seeds and growing some herbs. Even watering your plants each day can keep you grounded. Studies suggest that soil contains a microbiome with antidepressant effects and that gardening can improve mood as we're exposed to this soil bacteria as we dig it up.

Connect with your body

Adopting regular, daily or weekly routines for self-care can be very containing, creating consistency amid all sorts of stressful life events happening around you.

Looking in the mirror each day can actually remind you that you exist, so feel free to factor some reflective gazing into your daily routine, whether it's while applying moisturizer, shaving or simply brushing your hair. Studies have shown that being confronted with your reflection can have powerful effects, taking us out of our heads and into the immediate present.

For added effect, pay attention to the way your products interact with your hair and skin as you apply them.

Even simple acts like dabbing your neck with perfume or aftershave, plucking and exfoliating can get you in touch with different parts of your body and different sensations, so long as you enjoy them.

Playing around with smells, colors and textures in your hands will also engage your senses. Using a scented shampoo, treating yourself to luxurious scrubs, or smearing on the body lotion after a warm bath can be easy ways to do this.

If you're having a bath, light a candle, dim the lights, use bubble baths and salts or play some gentle music. This can all help regulate your breathing and heart rate, and give you a better night's sleep.

Take a breath

Remember to breathe. It sounds simple, but we can often forget to breathe when stressed, which can exaggerate and exacerbate our reactions. With your feet on the ground, take a deep breath as if you're drawing it up from the ground, through your feet into your legs. Keep breathing it up into your upper body. Hold for 5 seconds, then breathe out slowly. As you exhale imagine your breath leaving your body by flowing through your arms and fingertips. Repeat. By focusing on your breath, it can help get your stress response under control and help you figure out a calmer, more measured reaction to your situation.

Try a finger trace

A simple breathing exercise you can do at your desk or in the privacy of your bedroom is to trace the shape of your hand with a finger on your opposite hand, while you breathe in and out. Take a breath in as you trace upward toward the tip of your finger, then breathe out as you trace down toward your palm and continue until you've traced all of your fingers. Not only does this help you regulate your breathing, it helps to keep you focused on your body in the here and now. This can be especially helpful if you experience a lot of anxiety or if you struggle with a flight, freeze or flop response, because it gradually brings you back into your body on your own terms, increasing your feeling of control.

Clear your mind

Abandon all your thoughts and try to focus only on your surroundings. What can you see, hear, smell, taste and touch? Identify four things you can see, three things you can hear, two things you can feel on your skin and one thing you can taste. Pick out colors in the room you are sitting in, notice textures and different kinds of light. If somebody is with you, do this with them, telling them out loud what you can see, hear, taste and smell. The point here is that your senses are your best and easiest route back to feeling calm by coming out of your head and rooting yourself back in the present. This is incredibly helpful if you're having either a panic attack or flop response and is also a simple way to support someone else through theirs if they're struggling.

Speak it out

If you're able to, speaking your process out loud can be a powerful form of self-support. For example, saying: "My mind has gone blank, just bear with me" can actually prevent you from panicking or feeling stressed. Naming things out loud can paradoxically help them go away by taking away their power, freeing up some energy we're spending on fighting them. It also moves the responsibility to deal with it away from just you. This can feel counterintuitive or as though you're sharing your weaknesses, but in therapy circles sharing your humanity, especially in a group, is an act of leadership as it can set an example for others, making them feel comfortable to do the same thing.

The power of music

Music therapy research tells us our heartbeat can match the music we're listening to. It can slow it down or speed it up. So, if you're stressed and your heart is beating fast, music therapists recommend playing a song with low beats per minute (BPM).

In fact, music is proven to impact both our autonomic nervous system (heart rate) and limbic system (emotions). This is great news because it means we can use music to help us with stress. Here are a few ways you can use your Spotify playlist to soothe yourself:

1. Choose a song with a low BPM. Studies indicate that Mozart's "Symphony No. 40 in G Minor" is a great one for lowering blood pressure and heart rate.

2. Some therapists advise creating a playlist that helps you move through a journey of feelings. If you're feeling stressed and your heart is racing, start your playlist with something up tempo to match where you are—such as a disco track—and gradually bring it down. If you're angry, start with a song that matches your mood, then transition to the calmer place you'd like to get to.

3. Think back to the songs you were listening to at important moments in your life. Use these as a resource to allow different emotions to come up to the surface. You might find yourself shedding a tear or laughing. That's all OK.

4. Music psychologists have discovered your memories are most vivid around the age of 14. Think about what was in the top 10 at this time. Look it up if you have to. See if you can remember any songs that made you feel particularly calm or relaxed.

If anything is likely to trigger painful memories, consider doing these exercises with a therapist or a trusted friend.

Write a song

You might be used to writing your thoughts in a linear way in a diary (which can be helpful), but why not try mixing it up a bit by jotting down some lyrics or poetry. Now see if you can set your words to a piece of music—either something that you create yourself or a tune that you're listening to. Don't worry too much about getting it right, just allow it to flow. It will help you connect with your emotions, process them and begin to let them go.

Play an instrument

Maybe you're already a violin virtuoso or adept at piano or guitar. In which case, allocate an hour or so in the week to go for it without any goal or agenda. If you played an instrument in childhood that has since been gathering dust, consider revisiting it. Let yourself be free with it. In school, we were often made to play songs we didn't want to play or told to play perfectly. Now you can be free to forget all the rules. Let yourself be drawn to an instrument and interact with it in a way that suits your mood. Are you angry? Hit it. Are you feeling all twisted and tight? Make that noise on that violin. Let your expressions be matched by the sound you hear back. You may even wish to take up lessons or join a "music for well-being" group.

Let loose in a music studio or shop

Don't limit yourself to the instruments you already know. Maybe you were classically trained, but always wanted to learn the drums. Or perhaps you were a budding rock star, but never dabbled in the clarinet. Let yourself be curious about the sounds different instruments make and how they affect you. Spend some time holding them and getting immersed in the feel of them and just lose yourself in the moment. Head to a music shop or studio to see if you can access some unfamiliar instruments. Or find a music teacher who is willing to give you some lessons across a few different instruments, so you can try out a whole range. Don't forget your voice is an instrument, too. Research shows singing, whether alone or in a group like a choir, has huge effects on our emotional and physical health, increasing lung capacity, improving breathing and releasing pain-relieving endorphins.

Find your now

We can get so caught up in our thoughts and daily tasks, we can forget what's around us right now. Take a step back from whatever is happening and notice the obvious. Speak out loud if you want: "I'm in a room. I'm sitting on a chair. I'm looking at my computer." This gives you an outsider perspective of what someone would be seeing if they were looking at us. This can be a sobering way to get out of our heads and back into the present.

Create a support network

Now you know some basic grounding and breathing techniques, you can start to audit the support you have around you to help limit how tightly stress gets its grip on you. Support can mean anything from the people you turn to for help and advice, and formal therapy, to having things around you that help lift your mood and lead to calm. This can be music, sounds and smells, or can involve doing things you love such as going to the movies, reading or cooking your favorite foods.

The more support you can surround yourself with, the more of a buffer you will have to help you handle life's knocks. Brainstorm as many avenues of support as you can think of—from people to places to things—and go about putting them in place and making them part of your life.

A powerful way of doing this is to take a large piece of paper and separate it out into sections called people, places, things and activities. In the people section, write a list of names of the people you can turn to if you're in crisis. Under places, list all the rooms in your home that keep you calm or places you like to visit that evoke good feelings and memories for you. Under things, list all the physical items that bring you joy or calm. And in the activity section, write down all the things you know to help, like exercising, baking a cake or watching TV. Fold the piece of paper and keep it somewhere safe. Any time life feels too much, open it up, look at all the support available to you and think about how you can access it.

Release the pressure

Sometimes, we can over commit to making changes in our lives. They might seem a great idea to begin with, but the novelty can quickly wear off, especially if the weather is cold or you're not feeling well.

Instead of setting unrealistic targets, try to allocate some time toward those goals, whatever they are. For example, between 9 AM and 10 AM each day, dedicate an hour to sorting out your finances. It doesn't matter what you get done in that time, as soon as 10 AM comes make sure you end the task.

Or if a weekly exercise class is too much, for example, try walking around the block for 10 minutes each day. You might feel like increasing it as you get fitter or you might not, but by keeping your goals small you're more likely to stick with them.

Relax your muscles

When your muscles are relaxed, your amygdala receives a message that there's no threat. Notice if you're gritting your teeth or clenching your jaw and try to relax it. Then close your eyes and drop your shoulders. Make your arms go limp, so that if somebody were to pick one up and let go, it would drop right down again with a thump. Do a quick scan of the rest of your body, relaxing each part as you go. This helps to slow down breathing and heart rate and lower your blood pressure, triggering your body's relaxation response.

Harness your imagination

Imagine lying on a white sandy beach with crystal clear waves lapping around you or picture a sunset on a warm summer evening. Whatever your idea of serenity, take a few moments away from what you're doing just to close your eyes and picture this scene. Think of the colors, sounds and smells. Visualizations such as these are powerful ways to expand your ability to relax by regulating your breathing and heart rate as you focus on calm imagery. If you can get to an actual beach or watch a sunset, all the better.

Scan your body

With your eyes closed and feet firmly on the floor, scan your body slowly from your toes up to your hair. Take time to really notice each body part. Are your feet warm or cold? Notice the feeling of the ground beneath them and whether they're constricted by shoes or socks. Work your attention up to your ankles, shins, knees, thighs, groin, abdomen, chest, neck, shoulders, arms, hands, fingers and your face, including your lips, tongue, cheeks, ears, eyes and forehead. This activity focuses your mind on to your body in the present. As you pay attention, you will start to notice which parts of your body hurt or feel tense. Soon you will notice patterns around where in your body you habitually hold your stress. Maybe you frown a lot or clench your jaw. Understanding how stress shows up for you can help you in your journey to tackling it.

Get creative

Music isn't the only creative way to reduce stress. Cortisol is a hormone that naturally occurs in our body and the levels are high in people who are stressed. Scientific studies prove that cortisol levels significantly reduce in people who use art as a form of stress relief. In one study in the journal *Art Therapy*, 75 percent of people had lower cortisol levels after 45 minutes of making art, including drawing and painting.

Writing, dancing, watching films, reading, making things and building are also valuable. In fact, creative arts therapies like art therapy, dance therapy and drama therapy are used in a range of clinical settings to help with a host of physical and mental health issues. You can easily adapt some of the therapeutic techniques to fit in with your day-to-day life. You don't have to be good at dancing, drama or art to get the benefits, they're just natural forms of creative expression readily available to you. In the next few pages are some tips to get you started.

Try playing around with different types of creative outlet and find out which one most suits you. It might be making things, writing things down or role playing. Have fun learning what emotions come up and how you feel as you do them. You'll become more present in the moment and reconnect with the joy and freedom it should bring. This in turn can help you become more aware of your reactions to stress and help you to take back control.

Get artsy

Think of all the different art materials there are: paint, pencils, felt tips, charcoal, crayons. They each offer you a different experience when you use them. Notice the rules you place on yourself: When holding a delicate brush, do you paint cautiously? When handling crayons, are you free to crush them, break them or scribble less perfectly? This can give us powerful clues about the rules we're operating under and show what's causing us stress. We're then in a better place to challenge them. For example, you can challenge thoughts such as: "Making a mess is bad" or "I should be quiet when expressing myself."

Art can be a safe way of experimenting with breaking rules. So bash those crayons into crumbs, mix colors that don't match, use your hands to press paint on to paper or flick ink on to an old white T-shirt. If making a mess isn't your thing, the following pages hold more techniques to see you through.

Get groovy

There are many places to dance: in your room, in a class or on the dance floor. However you like to do it, dancing is a great way to express your feelings while getting your heart pumping and improving posture and flexibility. Try getting a group of friends together to go out dancing or take a partner to a salsa class. Some dances are more about precision and posture, like ballet, while others, such as disco or jive, are about rhythm and freedom of expression. It can also just be about jumping up and down on the spot to your favorite song and getting lost in the joy of that moment. Even tapping your feet beneath your desk can be something.

Free writing

Simply pick up a pen and write down whatever comes into your mind. Even if it's the same word repeated over again for a few lines, let it come as it wants to. You'll soon find yourself getting into a flow and eventually thoughts and feelings should start to emerge. Keep going until something starts to make sense. This can be a good daily practice to get into, as it puts you into a state of flow and helps you let go of trying to be perfect. Perfectionism can be highly stressful and contribute to burnout. Once you can learn to trust on paper, you can start to trust in other areas of your life. Choose what to do with your writing afterward—read it back, keep it in a journal, or rip it up and trash it. Pay attention to how it feels when you let your work go.

Meet your stress

Imagine your stress is a person. What do they look like? If you met them at a party, how would they approach you, what would they be wearing and what would they say? If you placed your stress at the dinner table opposite you, what would you like to ask it? Imagine what it would say back. What gender is it? What age? It can be helpful to get up and swap positions when you start talking from your stress's perspective. Sometimes giving your stress a voice and having a back-and-forth conversation in this way can give you helpful insights into what's really going on for you. And when you understand the root causes of your stress you can start to tackle it.

Document your dreams

When you're stressed, you might struggle to sleep or even experience vivid, lucid dreams. If you're able to recall your dream, write down the events of it in the present tense. For example, "I'm walking through my house looking at my dog, who is barking. Then I look out of my window and see a horse."

Try to remember as much detail as possible. What color was the front door you walked through? What kind of expression did the dog have on its face? Once you were outside, was there grass and what was the weather like? Were there raindrops on the windowpane? Pick out one detail of the dream such as one of the raindrops on the window. Retell the entire dream from the perspective of that raindrop. Try to avoid putting any interpretations on to your dream and simply describe what the raindrop sees. For example, "I'm on a pane of glass feeling the wind batter through me from behind. As I splatter on the glass, I see a room and a dog jumping up at a woman, wagging its tail." How does the raindrop feel?

When you're done, pick another aspect of the dream and repeat. In time, you'll start to access any feelings that are just out of reach and you will begin to build up a series of new perspectives to help you make sense of the dream in a way that's helpful. The idea is that all parts of the dream are parts of you and you can help widen the picture of your experience so that you've got more information and insight to play with. And with this greater self-knowledge you will be in a better position to deal with your stress.

Get organ-ized

Earlier in the book, you learned how to do a body scan, but now it's time to really get under your skin with an organ scan. Start by focusing in on your organs in turn. What's your stomach doing? Is it full or empty? Is your heart racing or does the beat feel regular and calm? Visualize your blood pumping around your body and your breath entering your lungs. How does it feel?

These parts of our body are working for us each day and we often forget they're there. Notice signs of hunger, thirst, tiredness or whether you need the toilet.

When we're stressed, we can forget to eat, drink and go to the toilet, which is why it's helpful to get in the habit of checking that you're meeting your physical needs, as this means you'll be in a better place to work on your stress levels.

Get walking

Whether it's a brisk walk, a long, winding hike, or just an amble around your local park for half an hour, getting some fresh air and your blood circulating makes a huge difference to your mental and physical well-being. Walking can be a great way to help you make sense of what's going on for you and to untangle problems in your mind, while also getting your heart pumping and releasing endorphins—feel-good hormones. Plus, a boost of vitamin D will also improve your mood and help soothe any stresses you are working through.

Swap Twitter for tweets

Put down your smartphone or step away from your computer and open a window. Allow the fresh air to wash over you, then close your eyes if it's safe to do so. Now spend a few minutes paying attention to the birdsong outside. How many different types of tweet can you pick out? If you can't hear any birds, choose a different sound to focus on. Can you hear any planes above you, the sound of car engines, the breeze through the trees, the sound of people talking or children playing? Really focus in on the nuances of the sound for as long as feels comfortable. Then gently open your eyes and take some deep breaths to center yourself again. This will help you feel grounded and take you away from your stressful thoughts, allowing you to gain perspective.

Get wild about life

You don't have to have a garden or live in a luscious neighborhood to get a sense for the wildlife that is living all around you. Instead really stop and take time to notice all the creatures you're sharing your space with. Maybe it's a procession of ants crossing the path in front of you or a tiny spider spinning a web in the corner of your window frame. Maybe you're lucky enough to spot a fox or squirrel in your garden, or a duck swimming on the river. Take a moment to watch the movements of these marvellous creatures and consider how life is constantly moving forward. As life happens everywhere, it will hopefully help you feel connected to the world around you and ground you, so that you feel stronger and more able to move through any stress you are experiencing.

Get sweaty

Clinical trials have shown that regular exercise can help stress, anxiety and depression. Aerobic exercise affects your metabolism, heart and how good you feel, reducing levels of stress hormones like adrenaline and cortisol in your body. It also helps to produce endorphins, the feel-good hormone, which elevate your mood, reduce pain and increase feelings of relaxation. Some exercises you can do by yourself include brisk walking and jogging, but if classes are more your cup of tea, try dancing, aerobics, Zumba, weightlifting in a gym or a weight-bearing circuit class. Long walks uphill can also have similar beneficial effects.

A recent study showed that regular weight training significantly reduces anxiety. This is believed to be rooted in molecular changes in the muscles and brain that help lift your mood. It also helps boost confidence as you can see your progress and also feel you have developed mental strength that can help you manage other areas of your life better.

But don't punish yourself if you can't make exercise a regular part of your routine or if you can't find a style of exercise you like. You're far from alone, and thankfully there are plenty of alternative routes to managing your stress.

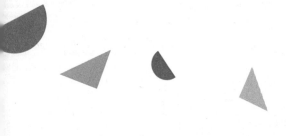

Find a furry friend

Research shows that spending time with animals has some seriously positive effects on our mood. If you already have a pet, you'll know that's true. Studies tell us that going to the zoo can really reduce stress, helping to lower our blood pressure and cortisol levels, and make us feel psychologically happier as we immerse ourselves in the experience. Why not take a day out to meet the penguins, feed the gorillas or watch the meerkats?

Alternatively, why not try dog walking or cat sitting, volunteering in an animal sanctuary or even walking down to your local park and watching the ducks? If you're very prone to stress or have a history with trauma, consider a therapy dog. Research shows that therapy dogs can increase your attachment responses, which in turn trigger oxytocin, the love hormone, helping to increase trust.

Meditate

Meditation is a way of training your attention on achieving a calm and positive mental state. You can make this as lavish or as simple as you wish. If taking a class helps, there are countless online and in-person options available to suit different budgets, but you can also keep it simple in a corner of your room.

Meditation master class

Remove all distractions, sit on the floor, close your eyes, notice your breath, scan your body and let your thoughts naturally disappear. Notice if your mind starts to wander. If it does, gently and with kindness, try again. You can choose how long you do this for, but if you're new to it, begin with 10 minutes, building up to half an hour. End with a closing ritual that means something to you. This could be giving thanks to the sunrise, making yourself a hot drink, blowing out a candle or listening to a song. The point is that it means something to you and honors the end of your meditation.

Laugh out loud

When it comes to reducing stress, laughter really is a great medicine. It gets your muscles moving, draws fresh air into your lungs, and boosts your mood and immune system. Maximize your exposure to laughter by making as much time as you can to fill your life with comedy. It might be watching your favorite sitcoms or a classic rom-com, listening to a podcast or going to see a live stand-up show. Or simply seek out your funniest friends. Spending time doubled up with laughter around people you love is one of life's greatest pleasures, and will help protect you from your stress taking over your life and happiness.

Make someone's day

When we're stressed, we're not always at our best. We can be irritable, angry, snap at others or lose control. The last thing we might feel like being is kind. Cognitive behavioral therapy research shows that changing our behavior can also impact how we think and feel about ourselves. Turning attention away from ourselves to make somebody else's day, such as performing an act of kindness for a stranger or a friend, can be one example of this. A compliment via text message, a lollipop in the mail, placing kind notes in books for people to find or leaving money in a vending machine for the person behind you can be a really simple way to give someone a boost, and in turn, lift your own mood. Try it and see how you feel.

Dealing with panic

Sometimes, you can feel so overwhelmed, it is impossible to think clearly. When stress gets to this point, you may feel panicked or like you're shutting down. This is a sign one of your five Fs is kicking in. Here are some useful strategies to help:

- If you're in fight mode, you're full of adrenaline. When it's safe, be aware of the effects of this on your body. If you're going to take on stress, try to factor in some self-care afterward, such as time off work or a night in if possible.
- If your pattern is to flee, place your feet on the ground and breathe deeply and slowly. Stick with your discomfort and allow it to pass. This will give you time to explore your options. What do you need to make this situation less stressful?
- If you freeze, allow the blankness in and don't try to change it. Paradoxically, this will make it pass. Once you experience this, you'll trust it more easily next time.

- If you're likely to black out or faint, try letting people know in advance so they can remove any hazards. Wear something you're comfortable in and have people around that you trust. If you're really struggling, therapy can be helpful.

- If you fawn, setting boundaries is important. Try to question your reaction. When you have some time after the event, ask yourself some questions, such as "What would be the penalty for saying no?" Write down two to five things that could happen, from the realistic to far-fetched. If each were true, what would that mean for you next? And if that happened, what next? Keep going until you find what's really driving you. You might see that doing something different won't end in disaster and the situation will be less stressful next time it occurs.

Put on your suit

You may remember a famous scene in the 1990s sitcom *Friends*, when Chandler panics on his wedding day and runs away. The thought of being married feels like too much to get his head around and this triggers his flight response. His friend Ross gently pulls him back to a place of calm by telling him to just put on his suit and not think about marriage. Once his suit was on, Chandler was in a better place mentally to contemplate the rest.

The key behind this success is in increasing the micro-levels of support that buffer you as you tackle a bigger challenge. If you're facing something that feels like an insurmountable challenge, imagine Ross with you. What's your version of putting on a suit? Do that, then come back to your original challenge. You'll notice how your experience of it changes and it should feel more doable and less stressful.

Something's got to give

If you have many things to sort out at once, it can be difficult to see the forest for the trees. Ask yourself if there is anything in this moment that can be dropped, pushed back or delegated to somebody else? It's not always possible, but sometimes you can push back on certain things to give yourself time and space to think. Are you the sort of person who needs to do the small things first before tackling the big challenges or do you get paralyzed with the small things because a big task is looming over you? Knowing how you work best will help you figure out what to tackle first and decrease your stress levels.

Play ball

If too many things are mounting up at once and you feel overwhelmed, this mental exercise can be helpful. Imagine a game of baseball with different bases. At each of these bases is one of your dilemmas to tackle. Visually run to the first base and spend time exploring that dilemma knowing the others will be dealt with later. Give yourself a time limit such as 10 minutes. Once your time is up, however far you've managed to get with your task, leave it and run to the second base and deal with the challenge there. After another 10 minutes, leave it and run to the third, and then finally the fourth base. Remember, once you've completed this circuit you can return to any of the other bases to finish anything that still needs your attention. This exercise can help you break down stressful tasks into manageable chunks and release some of your stress.

Practice yoga

Yoga is a spiritual practice encouraging flexibility, meditation and a mind–body connection that supports your well-being. The World Health Organization (WHO) points to its physical and mental health benefits, and suggests that regular yoga practice can help prevent and control diseases, such as cardiovascular disease, which prolonged stress can make us more prone to.

As well as tackling stress directly, yoga can reduce other issues that you might be living with as a result of stress, like heart problems. You can be any age and find a class to suit you, but you can also practice it at no cost in your own home. Look online to find a class that works best for you.

Be silly

As we get older, our lives can be taken over by responsibilities. That's no bad thing, but it means we sometimes no longer think about the things that used to give us so much joy in our childhood. Whether that's kicking leaves, skipping, playing with our friends, dressing up or spending hours learning to play the guitar, these were small, carefree moments that can still be incorporated into our adult lives if we allow them in. Throwing caution to the wind in the right way once in a while can feel so liberating. Below are ways to reconnect you to happier, more carefree moments in your life.

Play in the snow

If you're lucky enough to get some snow where you live, make the most of it and remember what it was like to be a child playing around in it. Harness that joy again by having a snowball fight, building a snowman and creating snow angels as you lie down in it. Remember, children don't mind if they get cold or wet as they know they can warm up with a hot chocolate after the fun is over! It's difficult to keep worrying about a work presentation when you're lost in the moment of crafting a perfect snowman face.

Burst a bubble

There's great joy and stress relief to be found in popping bubble wrap—it's the mix of the sound, the resistance in your hand, and the release of nervous energy and muscle tension as it pops that makes it so relaxing. If you have some on hand, pop away. Of course, with the reduction of plastic and attention to our environment, there are alternative ways of making this happen. Apps on smartphones or tablets now allow you to virtually pop, giving you a similar sensation. Or see if you can borrow a child's Pop It—a plastic fidget toy that has bubbles for you to push in— which is just as soothing as the real thing.

Hop, skip and jump

When was the last time you skipped? Chances are, it was when you were a child, before you grew up and forgot all about this joyful activity. Experts say that skipping is less stressful on your knees than running and burns more calories, too. You may feel a bit embarrassed skipping down the road on your own, so you might want to find a quiet path or take a child or willing friend out with you, so you can skip together. But you can also work skipping into your daily routine. Next time you take out the trash, why not consider skipping to the curb and back again? It will transform a dull chore into a fun one as well as lifting your mood and relieving your stress levels.

Have fun with foam

Next time you have a bath, reach for the bubbles and have fun. Alternatively, buy some party bubbles and place them by your desk at home. Blow some bubbles when the feeling takes you. Make shapes with them, watch them float away, or go ahead and pop them. This is visually appealing, a gentle sound to the ears and pleasant to smell. You might want to imagine that your stress is inside that bubble. Watch it waft away from you, burst and disappear. The act of taking in a deep breath before blowing will help you regulate your breathing and take in more air, increasing oxygen to your lungs, ultimately reducing stress.

Work on your well-being

The experts are right: how you treat your body matters. Sleep is vital to good health and exercise helps, too. Sleep regulates the stress hormone cortisol, and your pituitary gland releases growth hormone while you sleep, which helps with cell repair.

Exercise increases oxygen to the heart and lungs, keeping you stronger, fitter and healthier. It's understandable that when you're feeling stressed, finding the time and space to factor new habits into your routine isn't as simple as it sounds.

Changing your diet, exercise and sleep patterns when you're in the middle of major life-changing events can often feel like an extra chore added to the pile of everything else that leaves us feeling hopeless. Even thinking about what to do can feel more stressful than just getting on and doing it.

But you don't have to do it alone. In the following few pages, you'll find some creative exercises to help you work with this dilemma and free up some headspace for you to make any changes where you can. They can be done in your head, with a partner or friend or you can write them down.

Identify your vices

When you're stressed, what slips first? Is it your sleep, healthy eating, caffeine or alcohol intake, socializing, sex or exercise? Do you reach for the cigarettes, neglect household chores, binge-watch boxsets or ignore calls from family and friends? See if you can spot some patterns here. Then ponder on them. What function do they serve? Make a list. Why is it so unbearable to think about what you've got to do? Keep interrogating until you reach an "aha moment." If that doesn't happen right away, don't worry. The purpose of this exercise is to help you understand yourself a bit better before you rush to make changes. This will help you to make more lasting changes in the long run. The exercises on the following pages will give you some creative ways to unlock what might be going on for you.

Creative conflict

Usually, the vice you turn to is the thing you did the first time you found yourself in difficulty. Because it worked that time, you short-circuit to it when you're stressed. Whatever go-to vices you've identified on these pages so far, you wouldn't be turning to them if they didn't serve *some* purpose, even if counterproductive. If you want to get more in tune with what's driving your behavior, take a pen and draw a line down the middle of a piece of paper. On one side, write down all the reasons why you shouldn't be doing what you're doing. On the other side, respond with counterarguments.

Here's an example:

Eating chocolate	
I'm putting on weight.	Yeah, but it's comforting. If I eat it, it means avoiding feeling stressed for a few seconds.
It's not nutritious.	I know, but I crave the texture, which relieves tension.
It's ruining my teeth.	True, but it tastes good, and that makes me feel happy.

Give it a voice

Imagine the two sides of the paper as parent and toddler: the more a parent controls or ignores a toddler, the louder a toddler will cry. Start a conversation going between the two, as if they're actually talking to each other. Listen to the toddler voice: What is it trying to tell you? A creative way of doing this is to move from one chair to another, taking up the position of toddler and parent. If this feels like too much, try weighing up the two arguments with just your hands or get a friend or a partner to be the toddler voice countering everything you say. It should help you get an insight into why you're doing the things you're doing, which will help you to move away from any negative patterns.

Paws for thought

Imagine the parental voice from the exercise on the previous page as a top dog and the toddler voice as an underdog. Think about the way the top dog speaks. What tone does it adopt? What words does it use? How does it try to make you feel? What benefit does it get from getting you to do what it wants? Does it remind you of anyone? What does that reveal to you?

Do the same with your underdog. Why is it so resistant? What is it that the top dog can't seem to understand? What does it need the top dog to know? Who does the underdog remind you of?

You'll hopefully see that many internal battles have a lot to do with something unfinished with people in our lives. Rather than trying to keep fighting, can the top dog and the underdog find a middle ground?

Small changes equal big results

The great news is that there are so many small habits you can change or add into your daily life to help reduce the amount of stress you feel or limit the impact it has on you.

If diet changes prove too hard, try making easier changes around you. For example, decide to go to bed earlier than usual. This way you'll have less time to snack in the evening, so you'll effortlessly reduce your sugar and salt intake.

An early night might also help you to sleep better, especially if you enjoy a warm bath or read a book before you settle down for the night. Try to do something screen-free to stop the blue light messing with your natural melatonin levels.

Take regular breaks. Factoring in rest to your routine is essential to give you space and time for your body to recover and get perspective on any worries or problems. Don't wait until you're already feeling signs of stress before you take time off. Always have a proper lunch break, however busy you are, and take at least one full day off each week.

If time off just isn't an option, try adding some fun to your life. See your friends, do a grocery run, take up a hobby—anything that shifts you out of work mode. Don't try to make too many changes at once as you'll set yourself up for failure, which will just be another stressor.

If you're looking for some more simple changes to try:

- Drink some water before each meal.
- Download a fitness tracker to help you move more.
- Try stretching at lunchtime.
- See people you love, as this will release endorphins and boost you to tackle difficult tasks later.

Sort your sleep

The American Psychological Association tells us stress can seriously interfere with our sleep—not just how many hours we get, but the quality, too. This in turn increases our stress. Things like drinking caffeine and looking at computer screens just before you go to bed make the chance of sleep even less likely. The irony is these are the things we're likely to do when we're stressed. However, there are ways to tackle this cycle. Having a warm bath, using blackout blinds or an eye mask, switching off your phone and electrical items in the room can all help. So, too, can changing what you eat, drink and do during the day.

Quit sugar

Sugar makes our blood-sugar levels spike, increasing cortisol in our body, which in turn increases our feelings of stress. See if you can avoid putting sugar in your coffee and try to limit your intake of refined sugary foods, like cookies, sweets, chocolate and cake. You can swap them for naturally sweet alternatives like cinnamon, honey, fruit, or nuts including almonds and cashews. Don't forget to look out for hidden sugar in things like prepared sauces and breakfast cereals. You might find it hard at first and even experience sugar-withdrawal headaches, but keep going as it will be worth it.

Drink more water

Research shows that drinking just two cups less water than we should on any given day can trigger the release of stress hormones because our body is experiencing the feeling of dehydration. Aim to drink about eight glasses of water per day. If you don't like drinking plain water, try adding slices of fruit, mint or cucumber to get a natural flavor boost. Don't forget you can get your intake from hot drinks, too, but don't overload on caffeine. Choose herbal teas instead of tea and coffee.

Make it a multivitamin

Studies show that taking a daily multivitamin tablet alongside a balanced diet can significantly reduce stress and improve your alertness. Supplements containing higher doses of B vitamins are especially helpful toward improving your mood. A lot of these vitamins can also be found naturally in our diet, like omega-3 in oily fish, for example. The shelves in your local pharmacy or supermarket will be loaded with supplements, but a good quality multivitamin should do the trick. If you're worried about which to choose, or that you might need a boost of a specific vitamin or mineral such as iron, or have an allergy, speak to your health care provider for advice, and check first that what you're taking is compatible with any medication you're taking.

Pay attention

Have you ever noticed how many common sayings and phrases contain body parts? Things like "put your back into it," "keep an eye out" or "elbow grease." Usually the phrases we habitually say correspond to where in our bodies we store tension. Next time you feel an ache, think of a common saying that contains that body part. If you're feeling sick, what in your life are you sick of? If your back hurts, who do you want off your back? It should shed some light on what is causing you stress. Turn it into a game by writing down a list of sayings on some cards. With a friend, take turns to pick up a card and read it out loud. For example, "I can't stomach it." Tell your friend the things you can't stomach right now. Then swap. It will get your creative juices flowing and is a powerful springboard for deeper conversation.

Seek professional support

Many of the strategies in this book can be done in your own time at your own pace, but you might want to try something with more structure.

Keep in mind that some of the exercises in this book may be emotionally painful, opening up old wounds or bringing up things you may wish to explore further with somebody trained to guide you.

Having more structured formal support from a professional can be really helpful. This could be through counseling and therapy by qualified practitioners, alternative, holistic treatments, adopting the help of a personal trainer or nutritionist, seeing a doctor, attending support groups or using a helpline.

You don't have to wait until things are debilitating before you ask for help and support. In fact, research tells us that the earlier you spot signs of stress and get help, the less likely they are to develop into more chronic, complex issues.

If money is a factor, don't forget there are low-cost and free options available. Make an appointment with your health care practitioner for some advice and support, or look online for services in your area.

Visit your doctor

Depending on your personal situation, your doctor will advise you on whether to make some lifestyle changes. They may prescribe you medication, refer you to a specialist or make a referral for therapy. It can be helpful in advance to know what you're prepared to do. If you'd prefer to go down a therapy route instead of medication, let them know and vice versa. You know what's right for you. It might be worth researching your options before your appointment, so you feel prepared.

Call a helpline

There are many helplines available to support you, whatever issues you are facing. These are free and often accessible round the clock. They are staffed by volunteers who are trained to support you as and when you need it. Helplines can be useful when other services aren't available at the times we need them, for example in the middle of the night if you can't sleep.

There are two types of helpline. Those that offer a listening ear, without advice, to help you explore your feelings, and others that help signpost or give specific advice. Whichever you're after, don't be afraid to make use of them.

Seek out charities

Like helplines, there are hundreds of charities and community projects on hand to offer free advice and support for your particular issue. A simple search online can give you a list of them, but if you know a specific charity that could help, click on their website and follow the links to the support they offer.

Along with helpline services, many charities provide counseling, support groups, networking and events you can get involved with. They might even offer peer support by putting you in touch with people who are going through something similar to you, so you feel less alone.

Try therapy

Counseling and psychotherapy can be incredibly useful to help you work through stressful periods in your current or past life. They use talking to help you work through feelings, situations and events that have happened in your life. Consider counseling to see you safely through difficult periods, such as divorce, sexual assault, job loss or bereavement. Meanwhile, psychotherapy can help you take a deeper look back on your life to help you spot any unhelpful patterns you're getting into in order to cope. Psychotherapy can also support you with issues that don't always have one clear, identifiable cause, such as chronic stress. It can help you make clearer connections between your physical and emotional health. Counseling and psychotherapy are often done one to one with a trained professional, but you can have relationship and group therapy, too. There are many different approaches to talking therapy, which you'll see outlined over the next few pages.

Types of therapy

Most therapy happens weekly at the same time and day each week, but in some cases, sessions are more frequent depending on the style of therapy and your situation.

For example, cognitive behavioral therapy (CBT) is a goal-oriented therapy, usually carried out over a shorter period of time, and it works on the idea that our thoughts, feelings and behaviors are interlinked. By having a trained practitioner gently challenging our fixed beliefs about ourselves or what people think of us, and inviting us to change our behavior and notice what happens, we will change how we feel.

Neuro-linguistic programming (NLP) works with helping you to communicate in efficient and effective ways to get the most from your life in the here and now.

There are also creative art therapies where you can explore your feelings through music, art, drama or dance, instead of just through talking. You will have seen some techniques drawn from these in Part 1 of this book. They can be especially beneficial for anyone who is on the autistic spectrum, who has neurodiversity, or a neurological or learning disability.

If you're experiencing more of the flop stress responses described earlier as a result of complex trauma in your life, then consider therapies that address trauma-related stress.

In eye movement desensitization reprogramming (EMDR), a professional works with repeated eye movements to address negative thoughts, behaviors and feelings resulting from unprocessed memories without going into detail about the event. This can increase your ability to cope and function in everyday life.

Remember that there is no right or wrong therapy, only what works for you, and you may need to try out a few to see which works best. Always ensure your therapist is licensed, qualified to do the work they're offering and can show you their credentials when asked.

Psychoanalytic therapies

Psychoanalytic therapies focus more on your childhood development and early life experiences to help you understand how you relate to people today. This style of therapy is usually much longer term, with your therapist holding back a bit to give you a lot of space to talk. Generally, your therapist will give you time and space to talk and explore. They may occasionally reflect back or offer insight. Usually, they'll be fairly quiet, giving you space to work out what you need through talking. In long-term psychoanalysis, you may be lying on a couch with your eyes closed with your therapist behind you, but you should be able to choose whatever makes you feel most comfortable and relaxed.

Humanistic therapies

Humanistic therapies—such as person-centered therapy, gestalt, existential or transactional analysis—are less goal oriented and usually longer term (but not always). They involve deeper, two-way conversations between you and your therapist, helping you find meaning in your life and relationships, based on the point of view that you're influenced by the environment around you.

Your therapist will use their skills to help you find insights and answers by reflecting back what you're saying. They may help you notice connections or sometimes share with you what they're feeling as you tell them things. It's a powerful way to feel mirrored and seen. It may also include raising awareness of your body and you may try some creative exercises similar to the ones you've read in this book.

Get specific

Stress often goes hand in hand with other mental health issues that you may be experiencing. These could be anything from generalized anxiety, depression, obsessive compulsive disorder (OCD), an eating disorder, bipolar disorder or post-traumatic stress disorder (PTSD). Stress accompanies most clinically diagnosed mental health issues purely by how they impact your daily life. There are many variations on the standard cognitive behavioral therapy (CBT) to address your specific issue. These include acceptance and commitment therapy, dialectical behavior therapy, narrative therapy, compassion-focused therapy and, in the case of OCD, exposure and response prevention therapy (ERP). As for PTSD, the World Health Organization (WHO) recommends eye movement desensitization reprocessing (EMDR) as the first-choice treatment. In other words, there will be a therapy out there to help you as you work through your problems.

Hypnotherapy

In hypnotherapy, your therapist will explore goals with you and the techniques they're going to use, before helping you access a relaxed state and providing positive suggestions to help you deal with stress. You might feel tired or lightheaded afterward, though mostly calmer, but it's normal if you feel a temporary dip in mood, too. Think of it like a massage when you feel a bit sore or painful directly afterward before the benefits kick in. You cannot be hypnotized against your will and you're always in control. Always consult with your doctor first before undergoing hypnotherapy as it isn't for everyone, especially if you are living with certain psychiatric disorders.

Alternative therapy

The World Health Organization (WHO) considers traditional and complementary medicine as valid forms of health care that can be combined together depending on your issue. It defines traditional medicine, complementary medicine and herbal medicine in different ways and it's useful to know what they mean, both in terms of how they tackle stress and how they support your health as a whole.

Traditional medicine works to maintain your health and prevent sickness, while helping to diagnose, improve or treat physiological and emotional symptoms when they show up, through lifestyle changes, medication, surgery or physical therapies. It draws on the most up-to-date evidence, knowledge, skills and practices aligned with the beliefs of the different cultures around the world.

Complementary medicine (or alternative medicine) is a set of therapies that aren't part of your standard main health care system, but can be used alongside conventional medical practices to alleviate symptoms.

Complementary medicine includes:

- Massage
- Acupuncture
- Reiki
- Yoga
- Meditation
- Mindfulness
- Herbal medicine

You'll see explanations about each of these in the following pages and learn how they can work with stress. Some may suit you more than others, so keep an open mind and consult your doctor first if you want to try any of them.

Make it a massage

There are many types and styles of massage that can help with stress.

Aromatherapy uses essential oils from flowers and plants to treat issues. The scents of these oils have antiseptic or calming effects and a practitioner gently massages the oils into your skin to soothing music.

Swedish and hot-stone massages are equally as gentle but don't require oils. Instead, a therapist uses firm strokes to knead out knots and ease tension in your body. If you prefer more pressure, try deep-tissue massage for similar effects.

You can opt for reflexology, which uses gentle pressure on your feet; an Indian head massage, which focuses on the head and neck; or a shiatsu massage, which works with your whole body while you are fully clothed.

Thai massage is where you're stretched and twisted into positions to relieve pain stress, and improve circulation and flexibility.

Acupuncture

Acupuncture is the most common form of traditional medicine practice and is derived from ancient Chinese medicine. In traditional Chinese medicine (TCM), acupuncture relieves stress by encouraging movement of qi (vital energy) in your body. Your licensed practitioner will insert fine needles into specific parts of your body, which stimulate sensory nerves in the skin and muscles to produce endorphins, helping to relieve symptoms of stress.

Some other TCM techniques include cupping, moxibustion (burning dried herbs), tui na massage (combining massage and acupressure) and Chinese herbal medicine, all working with the concept of qi.

Reiki

Reiki is a Japanese healing technique. As with acupuncture, Reiki draws on the Eastern principle that vital energy flows through your body. Where acupuncture uses needles to target specific body points, a Reiki practitioner doesn't touch your body (or if they do, they use a very gentle light touch), but uses their hands to guide this energy to restore balance in your body, helping it heal and reducing stress.

Herbal medicine

Herbal medicine (phytotherapy) focuses on the health and balance of your body as a whole to restore its optimum function, or prevent or treat illness, through medicinal plants and herbs.

Phytotherapy uses natural plant remedies to promote good health and well-being, and is supported by some scientific research. Herbal medicines work to help the body heal itself rather than targeting illness specifically, and the herbs contain many ingredients to support your health in a number of ways at once.

Types of herbal medicine include Ayurvedic medicine, Chinese herbal remedies and Western herbal medicine. The Royal College of Psychiatrists has lots of reliable information on which herbal remedies are used for different mental health issues and how they interact with other drugs, if you're taking prescription medication, including their side effects.

Always tell your doctor or health practitioner if you are taking any herbal medicine before starting any new treatments.

Mindfulness meditation

Chronic stress can impair your immune system and make other health problems worse. For example, a consistent increase in heart rate along with elevated blood pressure can take its toll on your heart. While the insomnia, low mood and irritability that stress triggers can prolong chronic illness and depression.

Mindfulness meditation is a research-proven way to reduce stress. It works by lowering the stress response, influencing stress pathways in the brain and changing the activity in the areas of the brain associated with attention and emotional regulation.

Mindfulness-based stress reduction (MBSR) is a formal therapeutic intervention that encourages you to adopt a mix of yoga and meditation practices through structured courses and daily exercises that you can adapt and continue in your own time. These include mindful eating, walking or stretching, where you actively take in and observe your experience as it's happening.

Mindfulness-based cognitive therapy (MBCT) is another evidence-based intervention, combining

MBSR with CBT, which can be especially helpful if you're suffering with other mental health concerns alongside your stress, such as depression, anxiety or obsessive compulsive disorder (OCD). Speak to your doctor or therapist before trying anything new.

Mindful eating

- Focus only on your food, one piece at a time.
- Take in the look and smell of the food before you put it in your mouth.
- Experience what it feels like in your mouth, taking your time to chew properly and savor the flavor and texture.
- Notice it travel down your throat and how this leaves you feeling.
- Put down your knife and fork between bites to slow down your eating.

Complementary practices

There are many other holistic, spiritual, medical and complementary practices that can be used to tackle stress, including shamanic healing, crystal healing, homeopathy, cranial-sacral therapy, Bowen technique, chiropractic medicine, and other forms of energy therapy such as magnetic field therapy and light touch energy healing.

Depending on your religious and spiritual beliefs, as well as your personal attitudes to health, some may suit you more than others and are worth looking into. Like with all treatments, you should seek out well-trained, licensed professionals to deliver them. Know the credentials of your practitioner and the basics of what they're offering before committing. And remember that not all physical and mental health disorders are compatible with some styles of approach.

Always consult your doctor before trying out anything new and never stop or swap any current medication or treatment you're having for something else unless you've been given the green light from a qualified medical doctor.

Conclusion

We can't escape stress, but hopefully this book has helped you understand where it comes from and what you can do to prevent it from taking over your life.

Whether that's taking small daily steps toward a calmer, more peaceful way of life, or tackling a long-standing problem rooted in the past, you'll now have many of the tools and resources you need to cope.

Letting people know what you're going through, boosting your self-support and increasing the network of people around you will always help.

Return to this book any time you need a refresher, and feel free to adapt some of the tips and techniques to suit you.